Low (

The Ultimate Beginner's Guide To Low Carb Diet To Burn Fat + 45 Proven Low Carb Weight Loss Recipes

By Simone Jacobs

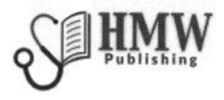

For more great books visit:

HMWPublishing.com

Download another book for Free

I want to thank you for purchasing this book and offer you another book (just as long and valuable as this book), "Health & Fitness Mistakes You Don't Know You're Making", completely free.

Visit the link below to signup and receive it:

www.hmwpublishing.com/gift

In this book, I will break down the most common health & fitness mistakes, you are probably committing right now, and I will reveal how you can easily get in the best shape of your life!

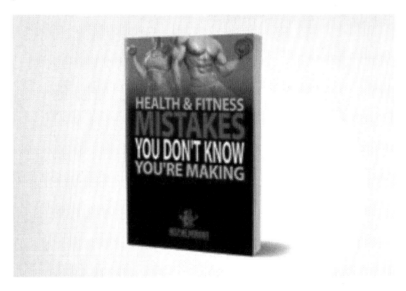

In addition to this valuable gift, you will also have an opportunity to get our new books for free, enter giveaways, and receive other valuable emails from me. Again, visit the link to sign up:

www.hmwpublishing.com/gift

TABLE OF CONTENTS

Introduction

I want to thank you and congratulate you for purchasing the "Low Carb Diet" book. This book contains proven steps and strategies on how you can successfully transition into the Low Carb diet. You will also discover how you can eat to your heart's content and still lose weight, as well as become healthier. Moreover, you will learn the advantages of reducing your carbohydrate intake. Furthermore, this book will also explain and reveal how to deal with the side effects. Lastly, we will also provide you 45 Low Carb diet recipes, which you can get started right away! Thanks again for purchasing this book, I hope you enjoy it.

Also, before you get started, I recommend you **joining our email newsletter** to receive updates on any upcoming new book releases or promotions. You can sign-up for free, and as a bonus, you will receive a free gift. Our *"Health & Fitness Mistakes You Don't Know You're Making"* book! This book has been written to demystify, expose the top do's and don'ts and to finally equip you with the information you need to get in the best shape of your life. Due to the overwhelming amount of mis-information and lies told by magazines and self-proclaimed "gurus", it's becoming harder and harder to get reliable information to get in shape. As opposed to having to go through dozens of biased, unreliable and untrustworthy sources to get your health & fitness information. Everything you need to help you has been broken down in this book for you to easily follow and to immediately get results to achieve your desired fitness goals in the shortest amount of time.

Once again, to join our free email newsletter and to receive a free copy of this valuable book, please visit the link and signup now: **www.hmwpublishing.com/gift**

CHAPTER 1: WHAT IS THE LOW CARB DIET?

More often than not, when we talk about diet, it means bland, unappealing food and meal choices, which does not inspire anyone to stick to healthy eating and living. Other foods are also ineffective that after months into it, the disappointment would make you quit.

You do not have to be disgruntled with your weight loss efforts anymore. How does crispy bacon and fried eggs in the morning sound? What about cream cheesy smoked salmon for lunch or butter-cooked steak for dinner? These meal choices do not typically look like dishes one would eat when on a diet. What if I tell you that not only can you enjoy many recipes as scrumptious as the one mentioned above, you would lose weight while eating them?

Sounds too good to be true, right? With the Low Carb diet, enjoying delicious meals while losing is not just a possibility. It will become your new healthy lifestyle habit. Who would not want to be able to eat almost anything and still be healthy and fit?

Eat Tasty Meals and Lose Weight?

Definitely! You will learn that with the Low Carb diet, limiting your carbs will still let you enjoy tasty meal options and even lose weight. This eating plan is deficient in carbohydrates, but it is fat and protein-rich, so you will not feel deprived and hungry.

Fat and protein-rich dishes? Isn't that bad? At first thought, it would seem that way. However, when you take a close look at this diet, it focuses more on healthy fats and lean proteins plus high-fiber as part of its plan. It's everything good that your body needs.

How Will the Low Carb Diet Help Me Lose Weight and Help Me Stay Healthy?

The Low Carb diet is a revolutionary weight loss and health plan approach that started many similar low-carb diet trends which emphasizes on restricting carbohydrates while focusing on eating healthy fats and lean protein.

Does It Work?

It does! In fact, it is one of the best low-carb diets, and various researchers show that it works. If you are a person who fills the day with lots of processed carbs, such as potatoes, pasta, and bread and does not eat many veggies and fruits, then this diet is what you need to start losing weight and become more healthy and fit.

In any diet plan, changing your eating habits and meal choices is always the first and hardest step. The tasty and many food choices of the Low Carb diet makes this first step easier than most of the other diets out there. Not only will this diet help you lose weight, it's a sustainable eating plan for a lifelong approach to a healthy lifestyle. You will not only lose weight; it will boost your energy and resolve specific health problems, such as metabolic syndrome and high blood pressure.

How Does It Work?

The primary emphasis of the Low Carb Diet is the right balance of carbohydrates, fats, and protein for optimal health and weight loss. According to this diet, the typical high-carbohydrate, low-fat diet is the cause of obesity and related health problems, such as heart disease and type 2 diabetes.

This diet stresses that you do not have to avoid trim excess fat off or avoid fatty cuts of meat. What's important is you control or limit your carbohydrate intake. Why? Eating too many carbohydrates, mainly white flour, sugar, and other refined carbs leads to imbalances in the levels of blood sugar in the body, which causes cardiovascular problems and weight loss. In that sense, the Low Carb diet emphasizes on restricting carbohydrates and promotes eating more fat and protein. Keep in mind, though, that this food is not a high-protein diet.

Track Your Net Carbohydrates

Carbohydrates are the sugars, starches, and fiber is found in grains, vegetables, milk products, and fruits. They are macronutrients, meaning they are one of the three main ways, besides of fat and protein, which the body obtains calories or the energy it needs.

While most of the other diets monitor the grams of fat or calories, the Low Carb diet does not require portion control or counting calories. What it requires is tracking your net carbs. When you limit the net carbs of your meals, your body will gradually learn to use and burn the stored fat of the body, which results in weight loss and better health.

How Do I Track My Net Carbs?

Net carbs are the total carbohydrate content (total grams) of food or dish, minus its fiber content (total grams). For example, 1 cup of cauliflower has 5.3 grams of total carbohydrates and 2.4 grams of fiber, giving it a net carb of 2.8 grams. Why do we subtract the grams of fiber? We do this because the body doesn't absorb fiber and it helps slow the absorption of carbohydrates.

When you count your net carbs per meal, you will start teaching your body to burn its stored fat and regulate blood sugar, which helps you achieve your ideal weight and optimum health, without making you feel hungry or deprived.

Keeping track of your net carbs intake will help you identify your tolerance to carbohydrates or the net carb grams that you can consume every day without losing weight or gaining weight. The more you learn about your carbohydrate tolerance, the better you can plan your meals for each day.

Do I Still Need to Exercise?

Aside from eating healthy, low carb meals, exercise is essential to weight loss and maintaining your ideal weight. So choose a physical activity that will suit your lifestyle and needs. Get moving and try to be active for at least 20 minutes or more every day.

The Phases of the Low Carb Diet

This low-carb diet has 4 phases. Depending on your weight-loss goals and need, you can begin your diet at any of the first three stages.

Phase 1: Induction

This step is strict. You will need to remove almost all of the carbs from your diet and eat just 20 grams of net carbs daily, getting them mostly from vegetables. Instead of getting 45-65 percent of your calorie need for the day from carbohydrates, you will only get 10 percent. During this phase, you will need to stick to the list of foundation vegetables, which are low-carb veggies, such as peppers, green beans, cucumber, celery, broccoli, asparagus, etc., and they should be the primary source of 12-15 grams of your net carbs for the day. Every meal should include protein, such as eggs, meat, poultry, shellfish and fish, and eggs. There is no need to restrict fat and oils during this stage, but you will need to remove most alcohol, nuts, grains, pasta, bread, sugary baked goods, and fruits during this phase. This phase will last for at least 2 weeks, depending on your weight loss.

Phase 2: Balancing

During this period, you will continue to consume 12-15 grams of net carbs from foundation vegetables and avoid foods with added sugar. You will slowly add some nutrient-rich carbohydrates into your diet during this stage, such as seeds and nuts, berries, melon, or cherries, legumes, tomato juice, and more vegetables. You will continue to lose weight during this phase and will stay in this stage until you are about 4.5 kilograms or 10 pounds closer to your weight goal. During this period, you can increase your daily net carbs to 25-50 grams.

Phase 3: Pre-maintenance

This is the stage where you can gradually widen the food range that you eat, including whole grains, starchy vegetables, and supplementary fruits. You can also add about 10 grams of carbohydrates in your diet every week, cutting back when you notice your weight loss stops. This is when you will discover the range of your carbohydrate tolerance. You will stay in this stage until you reach your weight goal. During this phase, you can increase your daily net carbs to 50-80 grams.

Phase 4: Lifetime Maintenance

After you've reached your weight goal, you will move on to this step, which will become your lifetime meal planning. You will have to maintain your daily net carbs between

80-100 grams.

How Much Weight Can I Expect to Lose?

During the first two weeks of the induction phase, you can lose about 6.8 kilograms or 15 pounds. This diet acknowledges that you will initially lose water weight. As you continue to phase 2 and phase 3, you will have a better idea of your carbohydrate tolerance, which will help you plan your meals so that you don't eat more carbohydrates than your body can handle.

CHAPTER 2: LIST ACCEPTABLE FOODS

So what can I eat? Well, to make it simple here is an accessible guide to the lists of foods that you can eat for each phase. I also included the net carbs of the most common food that you can choose from to plan your daily meals.

Phase 1: Induction – 20 Grams Net Carbs Daily (12-15 grams net carbs from vegetables)

You are free to enjoy most meat, poultry, and fish since they do not contain carbohydrates. However, refer to the list below to ensure that you are getting your 12-15 grams of net carbs in veggies as well.

All fish, includin g	All fowl, including	All shellfish, including	All meat, including	Eggs***, any style, including
Cod	Chicken	Clams	Venison	Soft-boiled
Flounder	Cornish Hen	Crabmeat	Veal	
Halibut		Lobster	Pork	Scrambled
Herring	Duck	Mussels*	Lamb	Poached
Salmon	Goose	Oysters*	Ham**	Omelets
Sardines	Ostrich	Shrimp	Beef	Hard-boiled
Sole	Pheasant	Squid	Bacon**	
Trout	Quail			Fried
Tuna	Turkey			Deviled

* Mussels and oysters are higher in carbohydrates, so limit your consumption to about 4 ounces each day.

** Some processed meat, such as ham and bacon is cured with sugar, which will add to carb count. If possible, void other meats and cold cuts with added nitrates.

*** Eggs are one of the most nutritious foods of nature. Hence, they are staples breakfast in the Low Carb diet. You can be creative with your eggs, adding onions, mushrooms, and even green pepper. You can also top a dish with feta cheese and sprinkle or garnish with oregano, basil, and other herbs.

Cheese, semi-soft, firm, full-fat aged, including (3-4 ounces per day)		
Cheese	Serving Size	Net Carbs
Swiss	1 oz.	1 g
Roquefort and other blue cheeses	2 tablespoons	0.4 g
Mozzarella, whole milk	1 oz.	0.6 g
Gouda	1 oz.	0.6g
cream cheese, whipped	2 tablespoons	0.8 g
cow, sheep and goat cheese	1 oz.	0.3 g
cheddar	1 oz.	0.4g
feta	1 oz.	1.2 g
parmesan, chunks	1 tablespoons	0.2 g

Salad Garnishes	Serving Size	Net Carbs
sour cream	2 tablespoons	1.2 g
sautéed mushrooms	½ cup	1 g

minced hard-boiled egg	1 egg	0.5 g
grated cheeses	See cheeses above for net carbs	
crumbled crispy bacon	3 slices	0g

Salad Vegetables (2-3 cups per day)	Spices	Artificial Sweeteners	Beverages	Oils and Fats (serving size: 1 tablespoon)

Free

sorrel	All spices, to taste, but make no added sugar	Sucralose, stevia or saccharine – 1 packet equals 1 gram of net carbs	Water (at least eight 8-ounce glasses per day including, mineral water, filtered water, tap water, and spring water	Walnut
romaine				
radishes				Cold pressed, or expeller pressed vegetable oils -olive oil is one of the best
radicchio				
peppers				
parsley				
mushroo ms				
mache				Sunflower*
lettuce				Soybean*
jicama			Unflavored almond/soy milk	Sesame
				Safflower*
				Olive oil
			Herb tea (no fruit sugar or barley added)	

17

fennel			Flavored seltzer (no calories and no aspartame)	Mayonnaise (no added sugar)
escarole				
endive				
daikon			Diet soda (made with sucralose or Splenda)	Grape seed*
cucumber				
chives				
chicory			Regular or decaffeinated tea or coffee*	Canola*
celery				
bok choy			Cream, light or heavy – limit to 1.5 fluid ounces or 3 tablespoons per day	Butter
arugula				
alfalfa sprouts				
			Club soda	
			Clear bouillon/ broth (no sugars added)	

18

* Always measure salad vegetable raw.

* 1-2 cups of caffeinated tea or coffee is allowed if desired and if you can tolerate. If you experience cravings or hypoglycemia, then do not use caffeine. If you have an addiction to caffeine, then the induction phase is the best stage to break the habit.

* Limit lime and lemon juices to tablespoons per day

*When using these oils, do not let the temperatures reach overly high. For sautéing purposes, use olive oil. For dressing salad or cooked veggies, use sesame or walnut oil – do not use them for cooking.

Foundation Vegetables

Vegetable	Serving Size	Net Carbs (g)
Alfalfa sprouts (raw)	1/2 cup	0
Artichoke (marinated)	1, each	1
Arugula (raw)	1/2 cup	0.2
Asparagus (cooked)	6 stalks	1.9
Avocado, Haas	1/2 fruit	1.3
Beet greens (cooked)	1/2 cup	1.8
Bell pepper, green, chopped (raw)	1/2 cup	2.2
Bell pepper, red, chopped (raw)	1/2 cup	3
Bok choy (cooked)	1/2 cup	0.4
Broccoli (cooked)	1/2 cup	1.8
Broccoli rabe (cooked)	1/2 cup	1.2
Broccolini (cooked)	3, each	1.9
Brussel sprouts (cooked)	1/2 cup	3.5
Button mushroom (raw)	1/2 cup	0.8
Cabbage (cooked)	1/2 cup	2.7
Cauliflower (cooked)	1/2 cup	1.7
Celery (raw)	1 stalk	1
Cherry tomato	10, each	4.6
Chicory greens (raw)	1/2 cup	0.1
Collard greens (cooked)	1/2 cup	1

Cucumber, sliced (raw)	1/2 cup	1.6
Daikon radish, grated (raw)	1/2 cup	1.4
Eggplant (cooked)	1/2 cup	2.3
Endive (raw)	1/2 cup	0.1
Escarole (raw)	1/2 cup	0.1
Fennel (raw)	1/2 cup	1.8
Garlic, minced (raw)	2 tablespoons	5.3
Green beans (cooked)	1/2 cup	2.9
Heart of palm	1 each	0.7
Jicama (raw)	1/2 cup	2.6
Kale (cooked)	1/2 cup	2.4
Kohlrabi (cooked)	1/2 cup	4.6
Leeks (cooked)	2 tablespoons	3.4
Lettuce, average (raw)	1/2 cup	0.5
Okra (cooked)	1/2 cup	1.8
Olives, black	5, each	0.7
Olives, green	5, each	0.1
Pickle, dill	1, each	1
Portobello mushroom (cooked)	1, each	2.6
Pumpkin, mashed (cooked)	1/2 cup	4.7
Radicchio (raw)	1/2 cup	0.7
Radishes (raw)	1, each	0.2

Red/white onion, chopped (raw)	2 tablespoons	1.5
Rhubarb (raw)	1/2 cup	1.8
Sauerkraut (drained)	1/2 cup	1.2
Scallion, chopped (raw)	1/2 cup	2.4
Shallot, chopped (raw)	2 tablespoons	3.4
Snow peas (cooked)	1/2 cup	5.4
Spaghetti squash (cooked)	1/2 cup	4
Spinach	1/2 cup	1
Spinach (raw)	1/2 cup	0.2
Sprouts, mung beans (raw)	1/2 cup	2.2
Swiss chard (cooked)	1/2 cup	1.8
Tomato (cooked)	1/2 cup	8.6
Tomato, small (raw)	1, each	2.5
Turnip (cooked)	1/2 cup	2.4
Turnip greens (cooked)	1/2 cup	0.6
Watercress (raw)	1/2 cup	0.1
Yellow squash (cooked)	1/2 cup	2.6
Zucchini (cooked)	1/2 cup	1.5

You will need to eat about 12-15 grams of net carbs each day from vegetables, which would be several cups, depending on the veggies actual carbohydrate content. One cup is about the size of a baseball.

Herbs and Spices

Herb/Spice	Serving Size	Net Carbs (g)
Basil	1 tablespoon	0
Black pepper	1 teaspoon	0.9
Cayenne pepper	1 tablespoon	0
Chives (fresh or dehydrated)	1 tablespoon	0.1
Cilantro	1 tablespoon	0
Dill	1 tablespoon	0
Garlic	1 clove	0.9
Ginger, fresh, grated	1 tablespoon	0.8
Oregano	1 tablespoon	0

Parsley	1 tablespoon	0.1
Rosemary, dried	1 tablespoon	0.8
Sage, ground	1 teaspoon	0.8
Tarragon	1 tablespoon	0

Salad Dressings

Herb/Spice	Serving Size	Net Carbs (g)
Balsamic vinegar	1 tablespoon	2.7
Bleu cheese	2 tablespoons	2.3
Caesar	2 tablespoons	1
Italian, Creamy	2 tablespoons	3
Lemon juice	2 tablespoons	2
Lime juice	2 tablespoons	2.4
Ranch	2 tablespoons	1.4
Red wine vinegar	1 tablespoons	0

> Any prepared salad dressing with no added sugar and has no more than 2 grams of net carbs per serving (1-2 tablespoons) is acceptable. Or make your own.

** If you decide to stay in Phase 1 longer for than 2 weeks, you may swap out 3 grams net carbs of some of the foundation vegetables with 3 grams net carbs of seeds or nuts. Do not let your foundation vegetable net carbs go below 12 grams.

The Transition at a Glance

To give you a better view of the transitions between each phase, here is a general guideline of the foods that you are allowed to eat during each phase

Phase 1: Induction –	Stage 2: Balancing –	Phase 3: Pre-maintenance –	Phase 4: Lifelong Maintenance –
20 Grams Net Carbs Daily (12-15 grams net carbs from veggies)	20-25 Grams Net Carbs Daily	50-80 Grams Net Carbs Daily	80-100 Grams Net Carbs Daily

Acceptable Foods	Acceptable Foods	Acceptable Foods	Acceptable Foods
Foundation vegetables	Foundation vegetables	Foundation vegetables	Foundation vegetables
Healthy Fats	Healthy Fats	Healthy Fats	Healthy Fats
Proteins	Proteins	Proteins	Proteins
Most cheeses	Most cheeses	Most cheeses	Most cheeses
Seeds and nuts	Seeds and nuts	Seeds and Nuts	Seeds and Nuts
		Melon, cherries, or berries	Melon, cherries, or berries
		Whole milk cottage cheese, ricotta, or Greek Yogurt	Whole milk cottage cheese, ricotta, or Greek Yogurt
		Legumes	Legumes
		Tomato juice	Tomato juice

	Additional Accepted Food	**Additional Accepted Food**	Additional fruits
			Whole-grains
	Melon, cherries, or berries	Additional fruits	Starchy Vegetables
		Whole-grains	
	Whole milk cottage cheese, ricotta, or Greek Yogurt	Starchy Vegetables	
	Legumes		
	Tomato juice		

During your transition between phases, remember to look out for your carbohydrate tolerance. The key is to find how much net carbs a day you need to consume without losing or gaining any weight once you have achieved your weight goal.

Chapter 3: Ketosis – Burn Fat and Lose Weight

Now that you are on your way to begin the Low Carb Diet, here is an accessible guide to acceptable foods for each phase.

The body usually uses glucose, derived from carbohydrates, for the energy it needs for the day, mainly to fuel the brain. When you are starting the Low Carb Diet, you are limiting your intake of carbs – usually found in many processed snacks, starchy vegetables, most fruits, pasta, bread, and sugar. Because your body is low of its primary source of energy – glucose from carbohydrates, your body is pushed into what is called a state of ketosis, meaning your body will now seek other sources of energy. It will start to burn fat for fuel, thus, encouraging your body to lose excess fat. When your body burns fat and uses it for fuel, it produces ketones, which becomes the body's primary source of energy. This is known as ketosis, and it is the key that makes the Low Carb diet a weight loss and health plan.

10 Signs of Ketosis

When your body is in the state of ketosis, it undergoes many biological adaptations, including a breakdown of fat and insulin reduction. When this happens, your liver will start producing large amounts of ketones to supply your brain with energy. However, it can be hard to determine whether your body is in the state of ketosis or not. Here are the 10 most common symptoms and signs of ketosis, both the positive and negative effects.

Bad Breath

This is a common side effect of the Low Carb diet and other similar diets once someone reaches full ketosis. Due to the elevated levels of ketone in your body, your breath will take on a fruity smell. The specific ketone that causes bad breath is acetone, which both exists in the breath and urine.

To avoid awkward social interactions, you will need to brush your teeth several times a day or chew sugar-free gum. Don't worry; this is not a permanent thing. The bad breath will go away after some time on the diet.

Weight Loss

This is one of the signs and symptoms that you want to achieve. When your body is in a state of ketosis, you will experience both short-term and long-term weight loss. During the first 2 weeks or phase 1, you will lose weight faster. However, most of the weight you shed during this stage is primarily water and stored carbs.

After the initial drop in your weight, you will consistently lose your body fat, as long as you stick to the diet plan.

Increased Ketones in the Blood

One of the trademarks of a low carb diet is the increase in ketones and the reduced levels of blood sugar in the body. As your body transitions from using glucose from carbohydrates as its source of energy to burn fat and use ketone as its primary source of power, the levels of ketone in your blood will increase.

If you want to know the level of ketones in your body, a specialized meter measures the beta-hydroxybutyrate (BHB), one of the primary ketones, in your blood. This is an accurate way of testing. However, it is somewhat expensive, so most people test once per week or every 2 weeks.

Increased Ketones in the Breath or Urine

Another way to measure the levels of ketone in the blood is using a breath analyzer, which monitors acetone, one of the primary ketones, in your blood when the body is in ketosis. This test is also accurate, but less reliable than the blood monitor method.

Also, first indicator strips can also be used to measure the ketone presence in urine. You can use this method daily. However, these pieces are not considered very reliable.

Appetite Suppression

This specific symptom is still being investigated, but many people claim that their hunger is decreased. Initial studies suggest that this may be due to increased vegetable and protein intake, as well as changes in the body's hunger hormones. It's also theorized that ketones may affect the brain in a way that it reduces appetite. So if you do not need to eat as often as before or feel full, you may be in ketosis.

Short-term Fatigue and Weakness

When your body first transitions to ketosis, it can cause fatigue and weakness. This symptom of ketosis may tempt you to quit the Low Carb diet before getting into full ketosis and reaping the various long-term benefits.

These symptoms part of the natural process. Your body has been running on glucose from carbs for a long time that it will take some time before it fully adapts to a new system. Achieving full ketosis does not happen overnight. It will take about 7-30 days.

So hang on tight. Don't give up just yet. Take electrolyte supplements to reduce fatigue. Your body will lose lots of electrolytes during the early phases of the diet since the body will eliminate lots of water and processed foods that contain added salt. Try to get 300 mg magnesium, 1000 mg potassium, and 2000-4000 mg sodium per day.

Short-term Decreases in Performance

Removing carbs as the source of energy can lead general tiredness, which results in decrease physical performance. This is caused primarily by the reduction of glycogen in the muscles, which provides the most efficient and primary source of energy for all high-intensity exercises.

When your body is in a state of ketosis, you will burn fat even more efficiently. Studies show that people on a low carb diet consume as much as 230 percent more fat than those who are not.

Increased Energy and Focus

When you are in the early phases of the Low Carb diet, you may experience what people report as feeling sick, tired, and suffer brain fog. Low carb dieters have termed this the "keto flu" or the "low carb flu."

Don't worry, as mentioned earlier; these symptoms are temporary. When your body has fully transitioned, your energy and focus will return and increase. It will take a couple of days for your body to adapt and start burning those fats for energy.

Digestive Issues

The Low Carb diet involves a significant change in the foods that you eat. You may experience diarrhea or constipation at first during the initial stages of transition. These symptoms will eventually subside. Just be mindful of the foods that cause digestive issues.

Insomnia

When you first change your diet and reduce your carb consumption, this may become an issue for you. This will usually improve after a couple of weeks. When your body has successfully adapted to the Low Carb diet, you will sleep better than before changing your diet.

When Does Ketosis Become a Concern?

The symptoms of ketosis will slowly disappear after the first phase of the Low Carb diet and shift out of ketosis. As you gradually increase your intake of carbohydrate to find your carbohydrate tolerance or carbohydrate equilibrium – the number of carbs you can eat without losing or gaining weight.

However, you must keep an eye on high levels of ketones. It can be toxic and can cause ketoacidosis, a condition that often occurs in people with type 1 diabetes whose blood sugar and insulin levels are not controlled. This situation is unlikely with the Low Carb diet plan. Nevertheless, if you experience symptoms such as dry mouth and skin, stomach pain, vomiting, muscle stiffness, headache, decreased alertness, rapid breathing, immediately consult a medical provider to make sure that your body is alright when undergoing ketosis.

Can I Still Follow a Low Carb Diet if I Am a Vegetarian?

It is possible to follow the diet when you are a vegetarian and even a vegan, but it will be difficult. If you are a vegetarian or a vegan, you will have to skip the first phase of the diet, which will limit your carb intake too much.

If you are a vegetarian, you can eat plenty of seeds and nuts and use soy-based food as your source of protein. You can also get protein from cheese and eggs. Coconut oil and olive oil are excellent plant-based source of fat.

Lacto-ovo-vegetarians can also eat cheese, eggs, heavy cream, butter, and other high-fat dairy foods.

If you are a vegan, you can get your protein from seeds, nuts, soy, legumes, and grains high in protein, such as quinoa.

If you are following a gluten-free diet, it will also be easy to stick to Low Carb diet. Foods with gluten are high in carbohydrates. People who follow the Low Carb diet usually eat less gluten than people on a standard diet.

The Low Carb diet is also a low-salt diet since you will need to stay away from packaged and canned foods as much as you can - foods that are also packed with added sugar, bad fats, and more carbs.

The Health Benefits of the Low Carb Diet

If you are still having doubts on whether to change your diet to Low Carb, then here are 10 proven benefits that will surely make you jump on the wagon.

Reduced Appetite

The single worst side effect of dieting is hunger. It's also one of the main reasons why most people feel miserable and end up giving up on their diet.

One of the best things about a low carb diet is that it instantly leads to appetite suppression. Studies consistently reveal that reducing carbohydrates and eating more healthy fat and protein results in eating much fewer calories – without even trying.

In fact, when researchers compare low-fat diet and low carb, it was found that they had to actively restrict the calorie intake of people in the low-fat diet to make the results comparable to those in the low carb diet.

On a Low Carb diet, you won't even have to try. When you reduce your carbs, your appetite will naturally go down. Hence, you eat fewer calorie.

Weight Loss

Studies show that reducing carb intake is one of the easiest, simplest, and most effective ways to lose excess weight.

People on a low carb diet lose weight faster than low-fat dieters, even when compared to dieters who are actively restricting their calories. Other studies show with a low carb diet; you can lose weight about 2 to 3 times more without getting hungry.

Weight loss is rapid, particularly during the first 6 months of the diet. Keep in mind, though, when you lose weight on the Low Carb diet, it does not mean that you can start eating the same old stuff. This diet is a lifestyle that you will need to stick to continually.

Lose Belly Fat

Not all body fat is the same. Where fat is located determines how it can affect your health and your risk of developing certain diseases. Our body has two kinds of fat – subcutaneous or fat under the skin and visceral or obese in the cavity of the abdomen. Visceral fat is the type of fat that tends to get embedded around the organs.

When you have a lot of belly fat, the visceral fat can lead to insulin resistance, inflammation, and cause metabolic dysfunction.

The Low Carb diet is very effective at reducing harmful visceral fat, which reduces the size of your waist. Over time, this will reduce your risk of developing type 2 diabetes and heart disease.

Decrease Triglycerides

Triglycerides are molecules of fat. Higher levels of triglyceride make you at risk of atherosclerosis or the narrowing and hardening atherosclerosis or arteries, which causes strokes, heart attacks, and peripheral vascular disease. High triglycerides also cause pancreatitis and fatty liver disease.

The primary cause of elevated triglycerides is overeating carbohydrate consumption, particularly too much simple sugar, such as fructose. When you reduce your carb consumption, it also lowers the levels of triglycerides in your body.

Increase High-Density Lipoprotein (HDL) Levels

There are 2 types of cholesterol, HDL or high-density lipoprotein and LDL or low-density lipoprotein. They are not cholesterols as most believe – calling LDL "bad cholesterol" and HDL "good cholesterol." They are, in fact, lipoproteins that carry cholesterol around in the blood.

LDL carries cholesterol from the liver to the rest of the body, while HDL carries cholesterol away from the body to the liver where it can be excreted or reused.

When you have high levels of HDL in the body, it lowers the risk of heart disease since cholesterol is efficiently carried to the liver. When you are on a Low Carb diet, you increase your intake of good fat, which increases the levels of your HDL.

When you are on the Low Carb diet, you increase your HDL levels and lower the levels of triglyceride at the same time, which effectively decreases your risk of developing heart disease.

Improves LDL Patterns

LDL or what most people call "bad cholesterol," which you learned earlier is not cholesterol, but a protein carrying cholesterol from the liver to the blood.

It is known that people with high LDL levels are more likely to have heart attacks. However, scientists have recently discovered that the type of the LDL matters – not all LDL is created the same. They have found out that the size of the particles is significant. People with small LDL particles have a high risk of heart diseases, while those with mostly large particles have low risk.

The Low Carb diet helps turn small LDL particles into massive particles, at the same time, reducing the number of LDL particles in the bloodstream.

Reduce Blood Sugar and Insulin Levels

Carbohydrates are broken down into simple sugars, mostly glucose, which is readily absorbed by the body. When you eat a lot of carbs, it elevates the levels of sugar in your body. To deal with high levels of sugar; your adrenal glands will produce hormones called insulin. To bring the glucose into the cells to burn it and use it as energy.

For most healthy people, the body quickly responds to minimize the spike of sugar to prevent it from causing harm. However, sure people develop insulin resistance, a condition where the body is unable to efficiently use insulin to burn and use glucose as energy, which leads to high levels of sugar and insulin in the body.

The Low Carb diet provides a solution for both conditions. When you cut back on your carbs, you will reduce sugar levels and insulin levels in your body at the same time.

Lowers Blood Pressure

High blood pressure or hypertension is a risk factor for many diseases, such as kidney failure, stroke, heart disease, and many others.

In a study published in the Archives of Internal Medicine shows that a low carb diet, such as a Low Carb diet, effectively helped obese and overweight people lose weight, many of which had chronic health problems, such as diabetes and high blood pressure.

Treats Metabolic Syndrome

When you consume too much fat, it can cause and lead to various conditions, such as high triglyceride and cholesterol levels, excess body fat, particularly around the waist, high blood sugar levels, and increased blood pressure. All these conditions occurring together is called metabolic syndrome, which increases the risk of diabetes, stroke, and heart disease.

You have learned earlier that a low carb diet efficiently resolves all of these conditions, thus it also effectively prevents and treats metabolic syndrome. With the Low Carb diet, you are hitting a lot of targets by just reducing the number of carbs you consume.

Therapeutic for Several Brain Disorders

It is known that the brain needs glucose to function. On the other hand, it is not widely known that some parts of the brain can only burn glucose, which is why the liver produces glucose out of protein when a person does not have any carbohydrates.

But the large part of the brain also burns and use ketones, which are formed when the body is not getting enough carbohydrates or glucose. It's a process where the body uses fat, particularly the bodies stored fat to fuel the brain.

This process has been used for decades to treat epilepsy in

children who do not respond to drug treatment. In many of these cases, a low carb, the ketogenic diet can cure epilepsy in children. In one study, it significantly reduces seizures and even stops seizures.

Currently, very low-carb or ketogenic diets are now being studied for other brain disorders, such as Parkinson's and Alzheimer's disease.

Chapter 4: How to Deal with Side Effects of the Low Carb Diet

If you are just starting on a Low Carb diet, you may experience some side effects while you are shifting from your regular diet to a low carb one. This chapter will focus on the common problems that you will encounter and their solutions.

Increasing your salt and water intake can solve the most common problems you will encounter. If you do this during the first week of your diet, then you will reduce the possibility of experiencing any of the problems enumerated below, or they will be minor.

Most Common Side Effects

Induction flu

This is the most common side effect most people experience with a low carb diet, like the Low Carb diet. During the first week of your diet, often on day 2 to 4, you may experience irritability, brain fog, confusion, nausea, lethargy, and headache. It mimics flu-like symptoms, hence, called the induction flu.

A headache is the widespread side effect of your transition to a low carb diet. You will also feel lethargic, tired, and unmotivated. Nausea is also common. You will even feel confused, experience "brain fog," and you may feel like you are not smart at all. Finally, you will also become irritable – this will be obvious to your friends and family.

The Cure: Salt and Water

Do not worry. These symptoms will usually disappear after a couple of days. The even better news, you can easily avoid these symptoms. They are often traditionally caused by salt-deficiency and dehydration due to a temporary increase in urine production.

You can add 1/2 teaspoon salt into a large-sized glass of water, stir until dissolved and drink it. Salted water can reduce or eliminate the side effects within 15 to 30 minutes. If it's useful for you, then you can drink it once a day for during the first week of your transition. You can also use bouillon or broth, such as chicken or beef bone broth for a better-tasting option.

Eat More Fat

When you are on a low carb diet, you need to make sure that you eat enough healthy fat to feel energetic or satiated. Otherwise, you will feel starved, hungry, and tired. Getting enough fat will speed your transition and minimize the time you need to spend feeling low when starting the Low Carb diet.

How do I get enough fat? There are many options, but when in doubt, add more avocado, butter or ghee, coconut oil, extra-virgin olive oil, and omega-3. These good fats can be found in seafood sources, such as sardines and salmon, some nuts, such as walnuts, seeds, such as flaxseeds and Chia seeds, and green leafy vegetables, such as watercress, spinach, kale, and Brussels sprouts) in your diet.

What if adding salt, water, and fat does not eliminate induction flu? The best thing to do is to hang in there. The symptoms usually go away within a few days as your body adapts to the Low Carb diet, and starts to burn fat.

If needed, you can add a bit more carbs to your diet to slowly transition into the Low Carb diet. However, this option is only a last option since it will slow down the process and will make weight loss and health improvement less obvious.

Leg cramps

This is also a common side effect when starting the Low Carb diet, or any low carb diet. It is usually a minor side effect when it happens, but it can sometimes be painful. This side effect occurs due to the loss of minerals, particularly magnesium, caused by increased urination.

How Do I Avoid It?

Drink plenty of fluid and enough salt. It will reduce magnesium loss and help avoid leg cramps. If needed, you can take a magnesium supplement. You can choose 3 slow-releasing magnesium tablets, such as Mag64 or Slow-Mag daily for 20 days. After 20 days, you can start 1 tablet daily.

If drinking plenty of fluids, getting enough salt, and taking magnesium supplements does not relieve the side effect, you can, again, eat a bit more carbs, keeping in mind that it will affect the impact of the Low Carb diet.

Constipation

When you are just starting on the Low Carb diet, your digestive system will need time to adapt, and you may experience bowel movement problems

Constipation is often caused by dehydration; so drink plenty of fluids. When you are on a low carb diet, you will excrete plenty of fluids from your body, which makes the body absorb more water from the colon, making the contents dryer and harder that causes constipation.

Likewise, you need to increase consumption of vegetables and other sources of fiber. This will help things in the intestine get moving, reducing the risk of constipation. You can add psyllium seed husks into your drinks for an utterly low-carb fiber addition.

If the solutions mentioned above are not enough, use milk of magnesia to relieve constipation.

Bad Breath and Body Odor

Earlier, you have learned that bad breath is a sign of ketosis. People often experience a fruity smell on their breath that they usually say reminds them of nail polish. This is the smell of acetone, a kind of ketone, which is also a sign that your body is burning fat, converting it to ketones to fuel the brain. Some people experience this smell is body odor when they are sweating a lot or working out.

Not everyone experiences ketone on their breath or body odor, and for many people, these side effects are only temporary and will often go away for about 1-2 weeks. As the body adapts, it will stop "leaking" ketones from sweat and breath.

However, for some people, these side effects do not go away, and it can cause a problem.

Like the previous solutions mentioned above for the other side effects, drinking enough fluid and getting enough salt can resolve it. You will feel your mouth getting dry at the start of the Low Carb diet when your body is getting into ketosis – this will mean that your mouth has less saliva to wash away the bacteria, which will result in severe breath, so you will need to drink plenty of fluids.

Second, you must practice a good oral hygiene. Brushing your teeth twice a day will into completely stop the keto smell, but it will prevent it from mixing with other scents. You can wait for 1-2 weeks - as mentioned earlier, this side effect is temporary and will go away.

Finally, if the term becomes a long-term problem and you want to get rid of it, the easy way is to reduce the degree of ketosis. This will mean that you will have to eat a bit more carbs, about 50 to 70 grams of carbs daily is enough to get out of ketosis. Of course, this will affect your diet. It can reduce weight loss and the health benefits, but for some people, a bit more carbs are still sufficient enough. Another option is to consume about 50 to 70 grams of carbohydrates a day along with some intermittent fasting. You will get roughly the same effect as a strict Low Carb diet minus the smell.

Heart Palpitations

During the first week on the Low Carb diet, it is also

common to experience a slightly elevated heart rate. Dehydration and lack of salt is too one common cause of your heart beating a bit harder. When there is a reduced amount of liquid circulating in your body, the center will pump slightly harder to maintain blood pressure.

The Cure

Again, drink plenty of fluids and get enough salt.

If Necessary

If drinking plenty of water and getting enough salt does not relieve heart palpitations, it can be the result of stress hormones released to maintain the levels of blood sugar. This is also a temporary side effect as your body adapts to the Low Carb diet, which will even usually go away after 1-2 weeks.

If the problem persists and your heart palpitations become bothersome – slightly increase the number of carbs you consume.

What If I Am Taking Medication for Diabetes?

Reducing the number of carbohydrates that raise blood

sugar will decrease the need for medication to lower it. Taking the same insulin dose before adopting the Low Carb diet can result in low blood sugar, which often results in heart palpitations.

When starting the Low Carb diet, you will need to frequently monitor your blood sugar and adapt or lower your medication accordingly. Keep in mind; you will need to do this with the assistance of a knowledgeable physician. If you are healthy or if you have diabetes using diet or Metformin to treat your condition, then there is little risk of hypoglycemia.

What if I Have High Blood Pressure?

High blood pressure improves or normalizes when you are adopting the Low Carb diet. You will need to reduce your medication because the usual dosage may become too high, which can lead to low blood pressure that also causes heart palpitations and increased pulse.

When you experience these symptoms, check your blood pressure. If it your blood pressure is low and under 100/70, then you should seek advice from your doctor to discuss reducing or discontinuing your medication.

Reduced Physical Performance

During the first few weeks of changing your diet to adopt the Low Carb diet, you may also experience reduced physical performance due to lack of salt and fluids and while your body is still transitioning from using glucose as a primary source of energy to burning fat.

Drink a glass of water dissolved in 1/2 teaspoon salt about 30-60 minutes before exercise will make a huge difference. However, there is no quick fix as your body shifts from burning sugar to burning fat. It will take a couple of months for your body to adapt and use energy fully. Nevertheless, adaptation will be faster the more you exercise while on the Low Carb diet.

Increased Physical Performance on the Low Carb Diet

While you may experience reduced physical performance while your body is still transitioning, the long-term benefits of the diet is an increase in physical performance when your body has completely adapted. Moreover, because your body uses stored fat as a source of energy, it will lighten your weight, which is a huge bonus for most sports.

Least Common Side Effects

Temporary Hair Loss

A dietary chance can cause temporary hair loss. Although rare, this can also occur in the Low Carb diet. When this does happen, it will usually happen about 3 to 6 months after starting the food, and you will notice an increase in the amount of falling hair when you comb or brush.

Do not worry. This is a temporary side effect, and the results of the hair fall will rarely be noticeable. After a couple of months, new hair will grow.

How Do I Minimize the Risk of Hair Loss?

Temporary hair loss is relatively rare, and you will never notice it when it does happen. However, it may help if you reduce stress during the first couple of weeks of the Low Carb diet. Also, get enough sleep, be gentle to yourself, and do not start an intense exercise program at the same time you start the Low Carb diet – wait at least a few weeks when your body is well on its way in transition.

Elevated Cholesterol

The Low Carb diet and other low carb diets improve your cholesterol profile. The classic effect of any low carb diet is a slight elevation of HDL or good cholesterol as people refer to it, which lowers the risk of developing heart disease. In particular, triglycerides become lower, and LDL particles become more substantial and fluffier.

However, there are also rare potential problems. A small number of people, probably due to genetics, who are on a low carb diet can have an unusually have a high LDL particle count, which indicates increased the risk of heart disease. There are recent cholesterol tests that can determine whether you have extraordinarily high LDL particle count.

If you belong to this small group of people, it is worth taking steps to correct and avoid potential risks.

Stop drinking bulletproof coffee (coffee with MCT oil, coconut oil, or butter) and do not consume a significant amount of fat when you are not hungry – this alone can normalize levels of cholesterol. Only eat when you are hungry and considering adding intermittent fasting. Consider using more unsaturated fat, such as avocados, fatty fish, and olive oil. Finally, think if you need to follow a strict Low Carb diet. If a more liberal or moderate diet, about 50 to 100 grams of carbohydrates daily, will work for you, then it will likely lower levels of cholesterol.

Lower Alcohol Tolerance

People who are on a low carb diet found out that it significantly takes less alcohol to get intoxicated. So be careful when during your first time you drink an alcoholic beverage while you are on the Low Carb diet. Most probably, drinking half as many drinks than you usually will get you drunk. Be prepared for it and don't drink alcoholic beverages more than you can handle. Always remember, do not drink and drive.

Potential Danger for Breastfeeding Mothers

An incident reported a breastfeeding mother who had been hospitalized for severe ketoacidosis. People immediately indicated that her low carb diet is one of the factors that caused her hospitalization. However, her ketoacidosis is not caused by her low carb diet.

She had been on a low carb, high-fat diet for about 6 years when the incident occurred. She also experienced stress during her second pregnancy and after her childbirth. She lost her appetite and didn't get enough energy and carbohydrates. She almost ate nothing while she was breastfeeding, which depleted her body of nutrients. To say that a low carb diet w what got her sick is not the complete picture.

Many women and mothers share stories about eating a low carb diet with great success and without any issues during breastfeeding. However, it is possible that a strict low carb diet can be too demanding during lactation when the body needs to produce carbs for breast milk. If you are on a tight low carb diet and you are breastfeeding, your body will have to provide more carbohydrates than women who do not breastfeed babies.

So far, there have been 5 cases of ketoacidosis during lactation, 2 of which are possibly linked to low carb diet while 3 are connected to starvation.

Although these cases appear rare, it is a good idea to be watchful on a low carb diet when you are breastfeeding. A great alternative is to consume a bit more carbohydrates, with more than 50 grams of carbohydrates daily. Keep in mind that breastfeeding consumes carbohydrates - do not take an unnecessary risk!

If you feel flu-like symptoms – headache, nausea, abnormally thirsty, weak, and sick – then you should significantly increase the amount of fluid and carbohydrates and immediately seek medical attention.

Keto Rash

This uncommon side effect occurs when you are on a low carb diet, but a few people do experience this, and it can be very annoying.

This itching sometimes referred to as "keto rash," can be troublesome and sometimes can disrupt sleep. The rash and itching are always almost symmetrical on both sides of the body and most often develops over the chest, armpits, back, and sometimes, neck.

What Causes Keto Rash?

There are many theories. However, there are a couple of common denominators. Itching usually begins soon after a person gets into ketosis and it usually stops 1-2 days after a person eats more carbs and move out from ketosis. The itching often gets worse during hot temperature or after exercising, and the usual place of the rash and itch are areas where sweat can accumulate. Ketosis sweat can contain acetone, which can be irritating at high concentrations. If we consider all of the above, then we can presume that the itching some people experience is caused by ketones in sweat, perhaps as it dries in the body.

How Do I Cure Keto Rash?

When the temperature is hot, wear comfortable clothes, so you do not sweat more than necessary and use air conditioning when needed. After exercising, it will help if you take a shower. If the itching becomes very troubling, you may want to skip exercise for a couple of days or choose an activity that does not produce sweat, such as a brief weight training.

If the solutions mentioned above do not resolve the side effects, you may have to exit ketosis and expect relief within 1-2 days. You can do this by eating about 50 grams or more of carbohydrates daily. To get most of the benefits of the Low Carb diet – at least for type 2 diabetes and weight loss, you can eat as much as 50 to 100 grams of carbs daily and add intermittent fasting.

Do not follow other suggested treatments you may read, like antibiotics or special creams. Antihistamines, anti-fungal creams, and steroids are not sufficient. The safest way is to exit ketosis.

Can I Try Ketosis Again?

The answer is yes, mainly if you feel great and get a lot of benefits from ketosis. The keto rash may stay away. Usually, people on the Low Carb diet only get it once, during the early stages of ketosis. Most people do not experience keto rash at all.

If you get rid of the keto rash by exiting ketosis, can you ever use ketosis again? The answer is likely yes.

Keep in mind all the advice above. If all else fails, then all you need to do is eat a bit more carbs, and the problem will most likely go away.

Chapter 5: Breakfast Recipes

Breakfast Rolls (Phase 1)

Serves: 6

Net Carbs Per Serving: 1 gram

Prep Time: 15 minutes

Cook Time: 15-30 minutes

Ingredients:

- 3 tablespoons cream cheese, light or regular, at room temperature

- 3 egg yolks, at room temperature

- 3 egg whites, at room temperature

- 1/8 teaspoon cream of tartar, at room temperature

- 1 packet sweetener

- Pinch salt

Directions:

1. Preheat the oven to 355F or 180C.

2. In a bowl, whisk the cream cheese with the egg yolks, salt, and sweetener until well blended.

3. In another bowl, beat the egg whites until foamy. Add the cream of tartar and, on high, speed, beat until stiff peak forms.

4. Gently fold the egg whites into the egg yolk mixture until just blended – do this very carefully to prevent the egg whites from breaking down.

5. Divide the batter, pouring it into greased 6-cup muffin top pan or silicone baking mat lined cookie sheet.

6. Bake in the oven for about 15 to 20 minutes.

7. Use to make burgers or sandwiches, or serve on its own with additional sweetener.

Notes: You can also make them at a lower heat, 300F or 150C for about 30 minutes.

Cheesy Ham and Bell Pepper Omelet (Phase 1)

Serves: 2

Net Carbs Per Serving: 4.6 grams

Prep Time: 15 minutes

Cook Time: 15 minutes

Ingredients:

For the filling:

- 1/2 cup cheddar cheese, shredded

- 1/2 cup ham, diced

- 1/2 tablespoon olive oil

- 1/3 cup bell pepper, chopped

- 1/4 cup onion, chopped

For the omelet:

- 4 eggs, large-sized

- 2 teaspoons olive oil

- 2 tablespoons water

- 1/4 teaspoon salt

- 1/4 teaspoon pepper

Directions:

1. Put the 1/2 tablespoon olive oil into a large-sized nonstick skillet and preheat over medium-high heat.

2. Add the onion and bell pepper; cook for a couple of minutes or until soft. Add the ham and cook until all the ingredients are lightly golden. Transfer the filling mixture to a bowl and set aside.

3. In a medium-sized bowl, whisk the eggs with the water, pepper, and salt until blended.

4. Put 1 teaspoon olive oil in the same pan and preheat over medium-high heat.

5. Pour in 1/2 of the egg mix and stir lightly using a spatula; cook until just set. Put 1/2 of the filing on 1

side of the omelet and top it with 1/4 cup shredded cheese. Fold over.

6. Continue cooking until the omelet is done and the cheese is melted. Transfer to a serving dish.

Repeat the process with the remaining egg mix and filling. Serve warm.

Cinnamon Soy Buttermilk Waffles (Phase 1)

Serves: 8

Net Carbs Per Serving Per Serving: 4.9 grams

Prep. Time: 20 minutes

Cook Time: 5 minutes per waffle

Ingredients:

- 1 cup soy flour

- 1 tablespoon baking powder

- 1 teaspoon vanilla extract

- 1/2 cup cold water

- 1/2 teaspoon baking soda

- 1/3 cup (75 grams) butter, melted

- 2 teaspoons ground cinnamon

- 3 eggs, lightly beaten

- 3/4 cup buttermilk

- 13 1/2 packets stevia sweetener

Directions:

1. Preheat the waffle iron following the instruction of the manufacturer.

2. In a mixing bowl, combine the soy flour with the baking powder, ground cinnamon, sweetener, and baking soda.

3. Add the butter, buttermilk, vanilla, and eggs; mix until well blended.

4. One tablespoon at a time, add in the cold water until you have a slightly thick but still pourable batter; discard excess water.

5. Pour about 1/3 cup batter in the center of the preheated waffle iron – adjust the amount according to your waffle machine.

6. Cover and cook on both sides of the waffle is slightly browned.

7. Repeat the process with the remaining batter. Serve warm on its own or with sugar-free syrup, or with fruits for Phase 3, if desired.

Soy Chocolate Pancakes (Phase 1)

Serves: 8

Net Carbs Per Serving: 4.9 grams

Prep. Time: 15 minutes

Cook Time: about 5 minutes per pancake

Ingredients:

- 1 cup milk

- 1 cup soy flour

- 1/2 teaspoon baking powder

- 1/4 teaspoon salt

- 2 eggs, large-sized, beaten

- 3 tablespoons (1 1/2 ounces or 42 grams) unsalted butter, melted

- 3 tablespoons unsweetened cocoa powder

- 6 tablespoons granulated Splenda

Directions:

1. In a mixing bowl, combine the soy flour with the cocoa powder, sweetener, salt, and baking powder.

2. Add the milk, flour, and eggs; mix until just smooth. Let the batter rest for 5 minutes.

3. Preheat a nonstick pan over medium heat. When the pan is hot, reduce the heat to medium-low.

4. Pour 1/4 cup batter into the pan and spread out. Cook until the bottom side is light brown. Flip and cook for 1-2 minutes more or until melted. Transfer to a serving dish. Repeat the process with the remaining batter. Serve warm with butter with some allowed fruits for phase 2 and 3.

Zoodle Stir-Fry with Parmesan and Bacon (Phase 1)

Serves: 2

Net Carbs Per Serving: 5.6 grams

Prep. Time: 15 minutes

Cook Time: 15 minutes

Ingredients:

- 1 green zucchini, medium-sized, julienned

- 1 tablespoon cooking oil

- 1 yellow zucchini, medium, julienned

- 2 tablespoons Parmesan cheese, grated

- 3 cloves garlic, chopped

- 4 slices bacon, cut into strips

- Grated lemon zest (from 1 lemon)

Directions:

1. Put the cooking oil into a large-sized frying pan and preheat over medium heat.

2. Add the bacon strips, cook until browned, and transfer into a bowl.

3. Add the garlic in the same pan; cook on medium heat until light brown.

4. Add the zucchini strips; cook for 1 minute. Return the cooked bacon and mix well.

5. Turn the heat off. Add the grated zest and grated Parmesan; toss until well mixed.

6. Season with salt and pepper to taste.

Jalapeno, Jack Cheese, and Soy Quick Bread (Phase 1)

Serves: 13 (2 slices each)

Net Carbs Per Serving: 1.5 grams

Prep. Time: 15 minutes

Cook Time: 35 minutes

Ingredients:

- 1 cup whole milk

- 1 tablespoon baking powder

- 1/2 cup soy protein powder

- 1/3 cup vegetable oil

- 1/4 cup vital wheat gluten

- 2 tablespoons butter, melted

- 3 eggs

- 4 ounces (113 grams) Jalapeno Monterey Jack cheese,

grated

Directions:

1. Preheat the oven to 355F or 180C.

2. In a large-sized bowl, combine the eggs with the milk, butter, and oil; beat well until blended. Mix in the grated cheese.

3. Sieve in the soy powder, baking powder, and wheat gluten; mix until just combined.

4. Pour the batter into a lined 8-inch baking pan and then bake for 35 minutes or until the bread is golden brown or a skewer comes out clean with inserted in the center.

5. When baked, cool the bread on a wire rack before slicing.

Soy Zucchini Muffins (Phase 2)

Serves: 12

Net Carbs Per Serving: 3.3 grams

Prep. Time: 15 minutes

Cook Time: 25 minutes

Ingredients:

- 1 1/2 cups soy flour

- 1 1/2 teaspoons baking powder

- 1/2 cup club soda

- 1/2 cup zucchini, chopped

- 1/3 cup granulated Splenda sweetener

- 3 eggs, large-sized

- 3/4 cup heavy cream

Directions:

1. Preheat the oven to 375F or 190C.

2. In a large-sized mixing bowl, whisk the eggs with the baking soda, heavy cream, and zucchini until combined.

3. Add the rest of the dry ingredients and whisk until well blended.

4. Spoon the batter into a piping bag and then pipe the dough into a lined 12-cup muffin pan until 2/3 full, leaving some room for the muffins to rise.

5. Bake in the oven for about 25 minutes or until slightly brown and a toothpick come out clean when inserted in the center of the muffins.

6. Remove from the oven. Transfer into the muffins on a wire rack and let cool.

Almond-Soy Cinnamon Mini Muffins (Phase 2)

Serves: 24

Net Carbs Per Serving: 1.3 grams

Prep. Time: 15 minutes

Cook Time: 20 minutes

Ingredients:

- 1/2 cup (4 ounces or 113 grams) unsalted butter, softened

- 1/2 cup ground almond

- 1/2 cup soy flour

- 1/2 teaspoon baking powder

- 1/2 teaspoon vanilla extract

- 1/4 teaspoon salt

- 2/3 cup granulated Splenda

- 3 eggs

- 3 teaspoons cinnamon powder

Directions:

1. Preheat the oven to 355F or 180C.

2. With a blender on MEDIUM speed, beat the butter with the vanilla and sweetener until fluffy.

3. Gradually add the eggs and beat until well combined.

4. Using a spatula, slowly fold in the mixed dry ingredients into the wet ingredients until well mixed.

5. Spoon the batter into a piping bag and the pipe the mixture into lined mini-muffin pan until 3/4 full.

6. Bake in the oven for about 20 minutes or until the middle is set. When baked, transfer the muffins to a wire rack and let cool completely.

Quick Almond Zucchini Bread (Phase 2)

Serves: 18 slices

Net Carbs Per Serving: 3.6 grams

Prep. Time: 20 minutes

Cook Time: 45 minutes

Ingredients:

For the wet ingredients:

- 1 zucchini, medium-sized

- 1/2 cup vegetable oil

- 1/2 teaspoon vanilla extract

- 4 eggs, large-sized

For the dry ingredients:

- 1 cup ground almond

- 1 cup soy flour

- 1 1/2 teaspoons ground cinnamon

- 1/2 teaspoon baking powder

- 1/2 teaspoon baking soda

- 1/2 teaspoon ground nutmeg

- 1/2 teaspoon salt

- 24 sachets OR 1 cup granulated sugar substitute OR to taste

Directions:

1. Preheat the oven to 350F or 180 C.

2. Coarsely grate the zucchini.

3. In a medium-sized mixing bowl, combine the wet ingredients and whisk until well blended.

4. In a large-sized mixing bowl, combine the dry ingredients and whisk until well mixed.

5. Add the wet mixture to the dry ingredients and mix until just combined and you have a thick batter.

6. Pour the batter into a greased and then lined 5x9-

inch loaf pan; smooth the surface.

7. Bake in the oven for about 45 minutes or until a
    skewer comes out clean with inserted in the center.

8. When baked, let the bread cool in the pan for 10
    minutes, remove from the pan, and let cool on a wire
    rack.

9. When cool, slice the bread into 18 servings using a
    serrated knife.

Breakfast Almond Bread Pudding

Serves: 2

Net Carbs Per Serving: 5 grams

Prep. Time: 15 minutes

Cook Time: 1 minute, 20 seconds

Ingredients:

- 4 tablespoons heavy cream

- 2 tablespoons butter, melted

- 2 packets Splenda

- 2 ounces ground almond

- 1 tablespoon flaxseed meal

- 1 egg, large-sized, slightly beaten

- 1 dash cinnamon

Directions:

1. In a small-sized microwave-safe bowl, mix the

ground almond, 2 tablespoons cream, 1 tablespoon butter, egg, flax seed meal, 1 packet Splenda, and cinnamon to taste until paste in consistency.

2. Microwave for about 1 minute and 20 seconds in an 1100 watt oven until the center puffs up.

3. Remove and immediately top with the remaining butter, cream, Splenda, and cinnamon to taste.

Breakfast Coconut Bars

Serves: 8

Net Carbs Per Serving: 3.7 grams

Prep Time: 20 minutes

Cook Time: 1 hour

Ingredients:

- 1 cup almond flour

- 1 cup heavy cream

- 1 cup Splenda

- 1 cup unsweetened coconut

- 1 cup water

- 2 scoops vanilla whey protein powder

- 3 teaspoons vanilla

- 4 eggs, large-sized

Directions:

1. Put all of the ingredients into a large-sized bowl and stir until well combined.

2. Pour the batter into a greased 13x9-inch casserole.

3. If desired, sprinkle the top with Splenda-sweetened coconut.

4. Bake for about 1 hour in a preheated 350F oven until golden brown.

Broccoli-Mushroom Quiche

Serves: 4-6

Net Carbs Per Serving: 8 grams

Prep Time: 10 minutes

Cook Time: 40 minutes

Ingredients:

- 5 eggs

- 10 ounces half-and-half

- 1/2 cup onion, diced

- 1 tablespoon olive oil

- 1 cup fresh mushrooms, minced

- 1 cup broccoli florets, cut into small pieces

- 1 1/2 cup Swiss cheese, shredded

Directions:

1. Sauté the diced onion, broccoli florets, and

mushrooms in olive oil and a glass ovenware or pie pan greased with nonstick spray – a 9x9-inch pyrex pan works well.

2. Beat the eggs with the half-and-half and cheese. Season to taste and pour over the veggies. If desired, you can add diced cooked ham.

3. Bake in a preheated 350F oven for about 40 minutes.

CHAPTER 6: LUNCH RECIPES

Asian-Inspired Beef Salad (Phase 1)

Serves: 5

Net Carbs Per Serving: 7.6 grams

Prep. Time: 20 minutes, plus overnight marinating

Cook Time: 1 minute

Ingredients:

- 4 ounces (113 grams) sliced water chestnuts

- 4 cups mixed salad greens

- 12 ounces (340 grams) beef sirloin steak, cut into thin strips

- 1/4 yellow bell pepper, cut into small pieces

- 1/4 red bell pepper, cut into thin strips

For dressing/marinade:

- 2 tablespoons tamari soy sauce

- 2 stalks scallion, finely chopped

- 1/8 teaspoon ginger powder

- 1/4 teaspoon curry powder

- 1/2 teaspoon granulated sweetener

- 1/2 teaspoon garlic, minced

- 1 teaspoon toasted sesame oil

- 1 tablespoons rice wine vinegar, sugar-free

Directions:

1. Except for the ginger and curry powder, whisk all of the dressing/marinade ingredients in a bowl until well combined. Pour 1/2 of the dressing/marinade ingredients over the sirloin strips; mix well to coat. Marinate overnight in the refrigerator.

2. Add the ginger and curry powder into the remaining dressing/marinades and mix well. Keep refrigerated and use as a salad dressing.

3. Put 1 tablespoon cooking oil into a large-sized sized

frying pan and heat until very hot.

4. Add the marinated sirloin strips and stir-fry for about 1 minute or until cooked medium done.

5. In a large-sized bowl, combine the salad greens, water chestnuts, bell pepper, and the stir-fried beef. Pour the dressing over and toss well.

Tomato Sauce, Onion, and Minced Pork (Phase 1)

Serves: 3

Net Carbs Per Serving: 6.2 grams

Prep. Time: 15 minutes

Cook Time: 30 minutes

Ingredients:

- 14 ounces (397 grams) minced pork

- 1/4 cup green bell pepper, chopped

- 1/2 tablespoons vegetable oil

- 1/2 cup onion, chopped

- 2 tablespoons water

- 3/4 cup sugar-free homemade ketchup

- Salt and pepper, to taste

- Sweetener, to taste

Directions:

1. Put the vegetable oil in a nonstick skillet and preheat over medium heat.

2. Add the bell pepper and onion; cook until lightly browned and softened.

3. Add the pork, season with pepper and salt, and cook until lightly browned.

4. Add the water, ketchup, and sweetener, mix well, and bring to a boil.

5. Remove from the heat and transfer to a serving dish.

6. Serve as a topping for spaghetti squash, zucchini noodles, or any low carb pasta.

Low Carb Diet Soup

Serves: 12 (1 1/2 cups per serving)

Net Carbs Per Serving: 4 grams

Prep. Time: 30 minutes

Cook Time: 32 minutes

Ingredients:

- 1/4 cup fresh basil, chopped

- 1 cup green beans, cut into 1-inch pieces

- 1 cup white mushrooms, sliced

- 1 tablespoon fresh garlic, minced

- 1 tablespoon olive oil

- 1/4 cup onion, chopped

- 1/4 cup sundried tomatoes, chopped

- 2 cups celery root, peeled and then cut into 1/2-inch cubes

- 2 cups water

- 2 cups yellow squash, sliced and then quartered

- 2 tablespoons red wine vinegar

- 4 cups cooked chicken breast, chopped

- 4 cups Swiss chard, chopped

- 4 slices bacon, cut

- 8 cups chicken stock

- Salt and pepper, to taste

Directions:

1. Put the olive oil in a large-sized soup pot. Add the bacon and cook over medium heat for 2 minutes.

2. Add the garlic, onion, mushrooms, and tomatoes; cook for 5 minutes. Pour in the water and chicken stock. Add the chicken and celery root; simmer for about 15 minutes.

3. Add the green beans, squash, and Swiss chard;

simmer for 10 minutes.

4. Add the red wine vinegar and season to taste with pepper and salt.

5. Just before serving, stir in the fresh basil.

Bruschetta Tomato Turkey Salad

Serves: 1-2

Net Carbs Per Serving: 4.4 grams

Prep. Time: 10 minutes

Cook Time: 15 minutes

Ingredients:

- 1 cup ground turkey

- 1 cup mixed lettuce

- 1 teaspoon basil paste OR a couple leaves fresh basil, finely chopped

- 1 teaspoon garlic, crushed

- 1 tomato

- 1-2 tablespoons olive oil

- 4-5 Kalamata olives, chopped

- Pepper

- Salt

Directions:

1. Dice the tomato and put into a small-sized bowl. Add the olive oil, olive, basil, garlic, and salt and pepper to taste.

2. In a saucepan, cook the minced turkey until browned. Add the tomato mixture and mix to combine.

3. Serve over a bed of mixed lettuce.

Chicken Taco Salad

Serves: 4

Net Carbs Per Serving: 8 grams

Prep. Time: 20 minutes

Cook Time: 25 minutes

Ingredients:

For the taco salad:

- 4 chicken breasts, boiled and then shred using a fork

- 1 yellow onion, large-sized, diced

- 1 head Iceberg lettuce

- 1 Can Rotel tomatoes, with green chilies

- 1 Can black olives

- Cheddar cheese, shredded

- Chili powder

- Cumin

- Guacamole, optional

- Olive Oil

- Sour Cream

For the homemade salsa:

- 1 large-sized can peeled tomatoes

- 1 medium-large-sized onion

- 1 small-sized bunch cilantro

- Garlic salt

Directions:

1. Pour the 2 tablespoons olive oil into a large-sized skillet and heat over medium-high heat. Add 1/4 of the onion and sauté until softened. Add the chicken, chili powder, cumin, Rotel tomatoes, and simmer for about 20 minutes, occasionally stirring.

2. Meanwhile, shred the lettuce and put in bowls.

3. When the chicken mixture is cooked, put on the lettuce,

heaping them on top. Cover with cheese, olives, remaining onions, and sour cream.

4. Put all the salsa ingredients into a blender and pulse until combined. Add to the salad – this will serve as the dressing. Enjoy!

Bacon Chicken Club Salad

Serves: 4-6

Net Carbs Per Serving: 5 grams

Prep. Time: 15 minutes

Cook Time: 30 minutes

Ingredients:

- 6 slices bacon

- 4 chicken breasts, boneless, skinless

- 2 cups cheddar cheese, shredded

- 1 cup mayonnaise

- Lettuce leaves

Directions:

1. Cook the bacon until crisp and then crumble.

2. Slice the chicken into cubes and cook thoroughly.

3. Put the chicken and bacon into an 8-inch cake pan.

Add the cheddar cheese and mayonnaise; mix to combine.

4. Bake in the oven for about 15 minutes.

5. Serve on top of a bed of lettuce. If desired, top with black olives.

Tuna Burgers

Serves: 4

Net Carbs Per Serving Per Serving: 3.5 grams

Prep. Time: 10 minutes

Cook Time: 10-15 minutes

Ingredients:

- 1 can (7 ounces) tuna, drained

- 1 teaspoon lemon juice

- 1/2 cup celery, diced

- 1/2 cup wheat bran

- 1/3 cup mayonnaise

- 2 tablespoons low-carb ketchup

- 2 tablespoons onion, minced

Directions:

1. In a bowl, combine all the ingredients. Divide the

mixture into 4 portions and form into patties.

2. Grease a nonstick frying pan with nonstick cooking spray.

3. Cook the patties until both sides are browned.

Artichoke Crab Cheese Puff

Serves: 1

Net Carbs Per Serving Per Serving: 4 grams

Prep. Time: 5 minutes

Cook Time: 20-25 minutes

Ingredients:

- 1/2 cup Sargento Pizza Double Cheese (cheddar or mozzarella);

- 1/2 cup Parmesan cheese, grated

- 1/2 cup mayonnaise

- 1/2 cup artichoke hearts, chopped (use canned - NOT marinated);

- 1/2 can (6-ounce) Lump, White Crab Meat, drained and patted dry

- 1 teaspoon garlic powder

Directions:

1. Grease a small-sized bakeware with nonstick cooking spray. Add all of the ingredients and stir well until mixed.

2. Bake in a preheated 350F oven for about 20-25 minutes.

Shrimp-Avocado Delight

Serves: 1-2

Net Carbs Per Serving Per Serving: 10.1 grams

Prep. Time: 15 minutes

Cook Time: 9-13 minutes

Ingredients:

- 3 ounces shrimp, peeled, cooked, detailed

- 1 avocado, medium-sized, cut into small-sized, bite-sized cubes

- 1 1/2 -2 tablespoons OR 3-4 cloves garlic, about already oven roasted in

- About 1/2 cup mushrooms

- Butter

- Garlic

- Lemon juice, to taste (about 1/2 fresh)

- Salt and pepper, to taste

Directions:

1. Melt butter in a nonstick frying pan. Add the garlic and mushrooms; sauté for about 3 to 5 minutes. Add the shrimp and sauté until warmed through, about 3 minutes.

2. Add the avocado, stir, and cook for about 3-5 minutes, keeping the texture non-mushy.

3. Squeeze the lemon juice over and season to taste with pepper and salt. Stir-fry until warmed through. Serve!

Bacon-Wrapped Scallops

Serves: 4

Net Carbs Per Serving Per Serving: 3.9 grams

Prep. Time:

Cook Time:

Ingredients:

- 1/2-3/4 pound bacon

- 1 pound sea scallops – do not use bay scallops since are too small

Directions:

1. Preheat the oven to 450F.

2. Rinse the scallops in cold water.

3. Cut the bacon into 3 sections. Wrap each piece of scallop with a slice of bacon and secure the bacon with a toothpick.

4. Put on a baking sheet and bake in the oven until the

bacon is crispy and browned.

Zesty Shrimp Salad

Serves: 3

Carbs Per Serving: 4.5 grams

Prep. Time: 13-15 minutes

Cook: 5-7 minutes

Ingredients:

- 1 pound shrimp

- 1 small-sized head lettuce

- 1/2 medium-sized cucumber, cut into bite-sized pieces

- 1 cup green bell pepper, cut into bite-sized pieces

- 1/4 cup Zesty Italian Kraft salad dressing

Directions:

1. Bring 1-quart water to a boil. When boiling, drop the shrimp in a boiling water and cook for 5-7 minutes. After 5-7 minutes, remove the shrimp from the pot

and let cool. When cool and peel. Toss with the salad dressing.

2. Add the rest of the ingredients and toss to coat.

3. If taking out for lunch, keep the greens separated from the shrimp. Just toss when ready to eat.

Cheese Ball in Ham Rolls

Serves: a lot

Carbs Per Serving: < 1 grams if using no carb ham

Prep. Time: 10 minutes

Cook Time: 0 minutes

Ingredients:

- Sandwich sliced ham (check for carb count)

For the cheese spread:

- 8 ounces cream cheese, softened

- 2-3 green onions, chopped

- 1/2 teaspoon garlic salt

- 1 teaspoon Worcestershire sauce

- 1 package thin sliced smoked beef (in the cheap little bags)

Directions:

1. Mix all the cheese ball ingredients until well combined.

2. Spread a cheeseball mixture in a piece of ham and roll. Repeat the process and serve!

Notes: You can keep a mixture of cheese spread in the refrigerator and roll with more ham as needed. This dish makes a quick lunch or snack.

Chapter 7: Snacks, Desserts, and Appetizers

Cinnamon, Coconut Milk, and Egg Custard (Phase 1)

Serves: 6

Net Carbs Per Serving: 4.3 grams

Prep. Time: 20 minutes

Cook Time: 35 minutes

Ingredients:

- 2 eggs, at room temperature

- 2 egg yolks, at room temperature

- 2 cups unsweetened coconut milk, at room temperature

- 1/4 teaspoon salt

- 1/4 teaspoon ground cinnamon

- 1/3 cup granulated sweetener

Equipment:

- 6 pieces (7-ounces) ramekins, lightly greased

Directions:

1. Fill a baking tray with water.

2. Preheat the oven to 300F or 150C.

3. In a large-sized bowl, whisk the eggs and egg yolks, mix in the sweetener.

4. Add the salt and cinnamon into the coconut milk; mix well.

5. Add the coconut milk into the egg mixture; mix well and then sieve the custard mixture into a jar or a measuring cup.

6. Pour the mixture into prepared greased ramekins until 2/3 full; cover with aluminum foil.

7. Cook in the preheated oven with a water bath for about 35 minutes.

8. Turn the heat off and let the custard stay in the oven for 10 minutes more.

9. Serve warm or chilled.

Bacon Wrapped Water Chestnut a.k.a Rumaki (Phase 1)

Serves: 24

Net Carbs Per Serving: 1.3 grams

Prep. Time: 20 minutes, plus 30 minutes marinating

Cook Time: 20 minutes

Ingredients:

- 8 slices bacon (cut crosswise into thirds)

- 12 water chestnuts (about 4 ounces or 113 grams), horizontally slice into halves

- 1/4 cup soy sauce

- 1/2 teaspoon molasses sugar

- 1/2 teaspoon curry powder

- 1 tablespoon granulated sweetener

- 1 tablespoon ginger, finely grated

Equipment;

- Toothpicks (presoaked in water for 1 hour)

Directions:

1. In a bowl, combine the molasses, curry powder, ginger, soy sauce, and sweetener; mix well.

2. Add the water chestnuts and toss to coat well. Set aside and let marinate for about 30 minutes.

3. Preheat the oven to 450F or 230C.

4. Drain the marinated water chestnuts; discard the marinade.

5. Roll 1 piece bacon around each water chestnut, secure with a toothpick, and arrange them on a broiler pan.

6. Bake in the preheated oven for about 10 minutes, turn, and then bake for 10 minutes more, or until the bacon is crisp.

Baked Buffalo Wings with Blue Cheese Dip (Phase 1)

Serves: 6 (1 chicken wing with 2 tablespoons dip)

Net Carbs Per Serving: 1.6 gram

Prep. Time: 20 minutes

Cook Time: 30 minutes

Ingredients:

- 6 chicken wings (about 1 1/2 pounds or 680 grams), halved and tips removed

For the marinade:

- 1 egg, lightly beaten

- 1 clove garlic, minced

- 1/2 teaspoon cayenne pepper, or to taste

- 1/2 teaspoon ground pepper

- 3/4 cup apple cider vinegar

- 3/4 teaspoon salt

- 6 tablespoons cooking oil

For the blue cheese dip:

- 2 1/2 tablespoons blue cheese, crumbled

- 1/4 cup sour cream

- 1/2 teaspoon garlic, minced

- 1/2 tablespoons lemon juice

- 1/2 cup mayonnaise

- 1 1/2 tablespoons scallion, chopped

Directions:

1. In a plastic bag or a large-sized bowl, combine all the marinade ingredients.

2. Add the chicken wings and toss to coat well. Set aside and let marinate for 20 minutes.

3. Preheat the oven to 450F or 230C.

4. Arrange the marinated wings into a lined baking pan.

Bake in the preheated oven for about 30 minutes or until cooked, basting 2 times with the marinade in between cooking.

5. Meanwhile, in a bowl, combine all the blue cheese dip ingredients.

6. Serve the buffalo wings with the dip.

Yorkshire Pudding (Phase 2)

Serves: 9

Net Carbs Per Serving: 3.8 grams

Prep. Time: 20 minutes

Cook Time: 30 minutes

Ingredients:

- 4 1/2 tablespoons beef or pork dripping, divided into 9

- 3 eggs, large-sized

- 2 ounces (57 grams) vital wheat gluten

- 1/2 teaspoon salt

- 1/2 cup soy flour

- 1 teaspoon double-action baking powder

- 1 cup whole milk

Directions:

1. Divide the dripping into 9 holes of a 12-cup muffin tin, about 1/2 tablespoon each.

2. Preheat the oven to 480F or 250C or the highest temperature of your oven or until the dripping is smoking hot.

3. Beat the eggs until frothy. Add the salt and milk; whisk until combined.

4. Sieve in the soy flour, baking powder, and vital wheat gluten; whisk until the batter is smooth.

5. Beat the batter again until frothy, light, and there are no more lumps, and a bit runny. If needed, add a couple of tablespoons of water if too thick. Transfer the batter to a jug.

6. Remove the preheated dripping from the oven. Continue preheating the oven to 375F or 190C.

7. Quickly divide the batter equally between the muffin cups with the hot dripping.

8. Bake in the oven for about 30 minutes or until puddings are slightly browned – do not open the oven until cooked. Serve piping hot.

Japanese Green Tea Meringue Cookies (Phase 1)

Serves: 4

Net Carbs Per Serving: 3.3 grams

Prep. Time: 15 minutes

Cook Time: 1 hour, 10 minutes

Ingredients:

- 3 egg whites, use 3-4 days old eggs, at room temperature

- 1/4 teaspoon cream of tartar

- 1/2 cup granulated sweetener OR 12 sachets

- 1 teaspoon green tea powder

Directions:

1. Preheat the oven to 250F or 120C.

2. Beat the egg whites until foamy. Add the cream of tartar and beat at HIGH speed until soft peaks form.

3. Gradually add the sweetener, spoon, while continuously beating. Continue to beat at HIGH speed until very stiff.

4. Gradually add the green tea powder; mix until combined.

5. Spoon the green tea meringue into a piping bag with your favorite tip. Pipe dollops onto a silicone mat OR parchment paper-lined cookie sheets.

6. Bake in the oven for about 1 hour and 10 minutes.

7. Let the cookies cool in the closed oven for 1 hour.

8. Carefully transfer into airtight containers. Keep refrigerated.

Pork Rind Nachos

Serves: 8

Net Carbs Per Serving: 3 grams

Prep. Time: 5 minutes

Cook Time: 4 minutes

Ingredients:

- 1 bag pork rinds

- 1 cup cheddar cheese, shredded

- 1 cup mozzarella cheese, shredded

- 1 tablespoon jalapeno peppers

- 1/2 pounds ground beef, browned

- 2 tablespoons sour cream

Directions:

1. Preheat the oven to 350F. Line a cookie sheet with foil. Grease with nonstick cooking spray. Spread the chips on the prepared cookie sheet, top with cheese

and ground beef, and put in the oven; bake for about 4 minutes or until the cheese is melted to your liking.

2. Top with the jalapeno peppers, sour cream, and your choices of toppings, such as guacamole and onions.

Faux Mac N' Cheese (IF)

Serves: 4

Net Carbs Per Serving: 6.2 grams

Prep. Time: 15 minutes

Cook Time: 15 minutes

Ingredients:

- 6 slices bacon, cooked

- 4 ounces sharp cheddar cheese

- 4 ounces cream cheese

- 4 ounces Colby jack cheese

- 2 tablespoons heavy cream

- 16 ounces cauliflower

- 1/4 cup green onion

- 1/2 teaspoon black pepper

- 1 teaspoon garlic, minced

- 1 teaspoon chicken bouillon

Directions:

1. Add the cauliflower to a microwave-safe glass dish. Cook in the microwave until fork tender.

2. In a medium-sized pot, add the cheddar cheese, cream cheese, cream, Colby jack, and minced garlic, and heat, continually stirring until smooth.

3. Put the cooked cauliflower into a food processor. Chop until all the cauliflowers are small pieces.

4. Put the bacon, cauliflower, chicken bouillon, green onion, and black pepper into the cheese sauce. Stir until mixed. Serve warm.

Low Carb Pizza

Serves: 16

Net Carbs Per Serving:

Prep. Time: 5 minutes

Cook Time: 30 minutes

Ingredients:

- 3 eggs

- 3 cups mozzarella cheese, shredded

- 1 teaspoon garlic powder

- 1 teaspoon basil, dried

- Your choice of pizza toppings

Directions:

1. Preheat the oven to 450F.

2. In a bowl, combine the cheese, eggs, basil, and garlic.

3. Press the mixture into a greased or parchment paper-

lined pizza pan or a cookie sheet.

4. Bake at 450F for about 10-15 minutes or until golden
    brown.

5. When baked, let the crust cool for about 15 minutes
    to firm. Flip the crust and dress the pizza with 1/4
    cup of low carb marinara sauce, 1 cup mozzarella
    cheese, browned and crumbled Italian sausage, sliced
    black olives, and onions.

6. Return to the oven and bake until the cheese is
    melted and the edges are browned.

Cheese, Avocado, and Flavored Tuna

Serves: 2

Net Carbs Per Serving: 6.8 grams

Prep. Time: 5 minutes

Cook Time: 0 minutes

Ingredients:

- 1 avocado

- 1 cucumber

- 1 small-sized tin flavored tuna

- Block cheese (your choice)

Directions:

1. Slice the cucumber to a reasonable thickness.

2. Put a slice of cheese on the cucumber. Add some avocado and then top with some flavored tuna. Enjoy!

Cheese and Bacon Stuffed Mushrooms

Serves: 15-20

Net Carbs Per Serving: 1.1 grams

Prep Time: 20 minutes

Cook Time: 10-15 minutes

Ingredients:

- 8 ounces cream cheese, softened

- 5-6 slices bacon, fried crisp

- 15-20 mushrooms, large-sized

- 1 onion, small-sized, chopped

Directions:

1. Preheat the oven to 350F.

2. Remove the stems from the mushrooms, reserving about 4-5 pieces of the stem. Clean the mushroom caps and set aside.

3. Chop the reserved mushroom stems and the onion.

4. Fry the bacon until crisp; reserve the bacon grease.

5. In the same pan where you fried the bacon, add the onion and the mushroom stems. Cook until softened. Drain the excess grease from the mushroom stem-onion mix and put into the bowl of softened cream cheese. Crumble the cooked bacon and into the cream cheese. Mix until well combined.

6. Divide the cream cheese mixture and scoop into the mushroom caps.

7. Put the cream-filled mushroom cap on a rimmed baking sheet and bake in the oven for about 10-15 minutes, and then broil until the tops are browned. Serve!

Notes: You can make these ahead of time. When ready to serve, just reheat in the oven.

Chapter 8: Dinner Recipes

Feta, Mixed Veggies, and Beef Patties (Phase 1)

Serves: 4

Net Carbs Per Serving: 1.3 grams

Prep. Time:

Cook Time:

Ingredients:

- 1 pound (450 grams) ground beef

- 1/4 cup feta, crumbled

- 1/2 tomato, medium-sized, chopped

- 2 tablespoons green onion, chopped

- 1/2 cup baby spinach, chopped

- 1/2 tablespoons fresh dill

- Salt and pepper, to taste

Directions:

1. Put all of the ingredients into a mixing bowl and combine until well mixed.

2. Divide the meat mixture into 4 portions and then form each part into patties.

3. Preheat a nonstick pan over medium-high heat.

4. Fry the patties for a couple of minutes per side until both sides are golden brown. Serve!

Grilled Salmon and Mixed Greens Salad with Italian Dressing (Phase 1)

Serves: 2

Net Carbs Per Serving: 6.9 grams

Prep. Time: 10-15 minutes

Cook Time: 10-15 minutes

Ingredients:

- 4 cups mixed greens

- 2 salmon fillets (5 ounces or 140 grams each)

- 1 1/3 cup tomato, chopped

- Salt and pepper, to taste

For Italian dressing:

- 1 tablespoon Parmesan, grated

- 1 tablespoon white wine vinegar

- 1/2 tablespoon parsley, chopped

- 1/2 teaspoon dried Italian seasoning

- 1/2 teaspoon garlic, minced

- 1/2 teaspoon Splenda sweetener

- 2 tablespoons mayonnaise

- Ground cayenne pepper, to taste

- Salt and ground black pepper, to taste

Directions:

1. In a salad bowl, combine all of the Italian dressing ingredients; whisk until well combined and blended. Set aside for about 5 minutes to let the flavors infuse.

2. Preheat the grill to HIGH.

3. Lightly season the salmon fillets with pepper and salt.

4. When the grill is hot, reduce the heat to medium-high. Put the fish on the rack and cook each side for a couple of minutes or until just cooked.

5. Add the tomato and the mixed greens into the bowl

with the dressing; toss well until coated.

6. Serve the mixed greens salad with the grilled salmon fillets.

Baked Salmon with Roasted Pepper Salsa and Bok Choy (Phase 1)

Serves: 1

Net Carbs Per Serving Per Serving: 3.9 grams

Prep. Time: 20 minutes

Cook Time: 10 minutes

Ingredients:

- 7 1/2 ounces (212 grams) salmon fillet

- 6 ounces (170 grams) bok choy OR your preferred green leafy vegetable

- 1/2 tablespoons olive oil

- 1/2 tablespoons butter, melted

- Grated lemon zest (from 1 lemon)

- Salt and pepper, to taste

For the sauce:

- 2 tablespoons homemade tomato salsa

- 2 tablespoons roasted red bell pepper

Directions:

1. Preheat the oven to 480F or 250C.

2. Season both sides of the salmon with pepper and salt.

3. In a baking dish, combine the butter and the olive oil. Add the seasoned salmon and coat well with the butter mixture.

4. Bake the fish in the oven for about 5 minutes, flip, and continue baking for 5 minutes or until the salmon fillets are just cooked.

5. Transfer the cooked fish to a plate and tent with foil to keep warm.

6. In the same baking dish, add the bok choy or preferred greens and the lemon zest. Coat with oil and warm the vegetables in the oven.

7. Put all the sauce ingredients in a blender and blend

until well combined.

8. Serve the cooked veggie with the salmon and the salsa sauce.

Garlic-Lemon Chicken

Serves: 3-4

Net Carbs Per Serving: 0.6 grams

Prep. Time: 10 minutes

Cook Time: 4 hours on HIGH or for 8 HOURS on low

Ingredients:

- 3-4 Chicken Breasts, large-sized, cut into halves

- 3/4 cup chicken stock

- 1/4 teaspoon salt, per chicken breast

- 1/4 teaspoon pepper, per chicken breast

- 1/2-1 teaspoon oregano, per chicken breast

- 1 teaspoon garlic, minced

- 1 lemon

- 3-4 tablespoons butter

Directions:

1. Take a re-sealable plastic bag, like a Ziploc bag, and using the "shake-and-bake" method, put the chicken in the bag. Add the oregano, pepper, and salt – to get the best result, place 2 chicken breasts into the bag and then add corresponding oregano, pepper, and salt. Repeat the process with the remaining chicken and spices.

2. Put 1 tablespoon of butter per chicken in a nonstick skillet. Put the chicken and cook until both sides are browned and then transfer the chicken to a slow cooker and crockpot.

3. When all the chicken is browned and in the slow cooker/crockpot, add the chicken stock, lemon juice, and garlic into the skillet. Scrape any browned bits from the skillet and bring to a boil. When boiling, turn the heat off and then pour the mixture into the crockpot.

4. Cook for 4 hours on HIGH or 8 HOURS on low. Serve with cauliflower.

Meatloaf

Serves: 7

Net Carbs Per Serving: 6.3 grams

Prep. Time: 15 minutes

Cook Time: 30-35 minutes or 45-60 minutes

Ingredients:

For the meatloaf:

- 2 pounds ground beef

- 2 eggs

- 2 cloves garlic, minced

- 1/3 cups ketchup, low carb

- 1/2 teaspoons pepper, or to taste

- 1 teaspoon salt, or to taste

- 1 teaspoon dried cilantro OR 2 tablespoons fresh cilantro

- 1 tablespoon Worcestershire sauce

- 1 tablespoon chili powder

- 4 ounces cheddar cheese, shredded

For the topping:

- 1 1/2 teaspoons Splenda granular OR equivalent liquid Splenda

- 1/4 cups ketchup, low carb

- 1/4 teaspoons blackstrap molasses

Directions:

1. In a large-sized bowl, mix all of the meatloaf ingredients until thoroughly mixed.

2. In a small-sized bowl, mix all of the topping ingredients.

3. Put the meat mixture into a greased loaf pan or shape into 6 mini loaves and put into a foil-lined 9x13-inch baking pan.

4. Spread or brush the top with the topping mixture.

5. Bake for about 375F for about 45-60 minutes for single large-sized loaf or about 30-35 minutes for mini loaves or until the internal temperature reaches 140-145F.

Cauliflower Crust Pizza

Serves: 4

Net Carbs Per Serving: 10 grams

Prep. Time: 30 minutes

Cook Time: 30 minutes

Ingredients:

- 1 cup chicken breast OR thigh, cooked and shredded

- 1 cup pumpkin, cubed

- 1 egg

- 1 pinch chili flakes, optional

- 1 pinch pepper

- 1 pinch salt

- 1 shallot, chopped

- 1/4 cup bell pepper, chopped

- 1/4 cup mozzarella, grated

- 1/4 cup onion, chopped

- 1/4 cup tomato, chopped, for topping

- 1/4 cup tomato, finely chopped, for salsa

- 400 grams cauliflower florets

- 50 grams parmesan, finely grated

Directions:

1. Preheat a conventional oven to 230C or a fan-forced oven to 210C.

2. Put the cauliflower into a food processor; process until fine. Transfer to a microwavable bowl, cover, and microwave for 10 minutes on HIGH or until very tender.

3. Drain through a fine mesh sifter, pressing down well using a wooden spoon to squeeze out excess liquid.

4. Lightly whisk the egg in a bowl. Add the cauliflower and 1/2 of the parmesan; combine until mixed.

5. Line a 30-cm, round-shaped pizza tray with baking

paper. Evenly spread the cauliflower mix on the plate, firmly pressing. Bake in the oven for about 20 minutes or until golden brown.

6. Meanwhile, put the pumpkin cubes in a microwavable container; microwave for about 5 to 7 minutes on HIGH or until soft. When cooked and mushy, mixed in a food processor or mash. When the pumpkin is mashed, add the finely chopped tomato, salt, pepper, and, if desired, chili flakes.

7. When the cauliflower crust is baked, take out from the oven. Evenly spread the pumpkin mix on the crust. Top with the mozzarella cheese, shredded chicken, shallots, onion, bell pepper, and remaining tomatoes. Sprinkle with the top with the remaining parmesan cheese.

8. Return to the oven and bake for about 7 minutes or until the cheese is melted.

Turkey and Shrimp Feta Alfredo

Serves: 3

Net Carbs Per Serving: 6.1 grams

Prep. Time: 30 minutes

Cook Time: 30 minutes

Ingredients:

- 8 ounces fresh shrimp

- 4 tablespoons heavy whipping cream

- 4 tablespoons feta cheese

- 4 ounces turkey or pork or chicken

- 2 teaspoons pepper

- 2 tablespoons of butter

- 1 teaspoon paprika

- 1 teaspoon granulated garlic

- 1 tablespoons parsley

- 1 cup vanilla soy slender

- 1 cup spaghetti squash, cooked

- 1 cup fresh mushrooms

- 1 cup fresh broccoli, chopped

Directions:

For the spaghetti squash:

1. Cut the spaghetti squash into halves.

2. Remove the strings and seeds from the center of the squash. Put a paper napkin on the top of the squash and microwave for 15 minutes or until cooked. Check after 15 minutes – you should be able to scrape the spaghetti squash using a fork, separating into strands.

3. Remove the spaghetti squash from the microwave. Measure 1 cup worth of spaghetti squash and set aside. Refrigerate the excess spaghetti squash.

For the feta Alfredo sauce:

1. Put the soy milk and whipping cream into a pan; bring to a low boil.

2. Add the feta and, with a whip, whip to mix. The cream should thicken a bit. Turn the heat off; set aside.

For the rest of the ingredients:

1. While the spaghetti squash is cooking.

2. Put 2 tablespoons butter into a skillet. Add the mushrooms and broccoli, cover and cook for about 5 to 10 minutes.

3. Add the cooked turkey and shrimp; cook for 5 minutes.

4. Add all the seasoning and the spaghetti squash. Mix well.

5. Pour the feta sauce over the meat and veggies; mix well.

6. Simmer for about 2-5 minutes.

Garlic and Lemon Butter Fish

Serves: 4

Net Carbs Per Serving: 16 grams

Prep. Time: 15 minutes

Cook Time: 12 minutes

Ingredients:

- 4 white fish fillets, your choice (cod, halibut, etc.)

- 4 garlic cloves, minced

- 2 tablespoons fresh parsley, minced

- 1/4 cup ghee, melted

- 1 lemon, zested and juiced

- 1 lemon, sliced

- Sea salt and freshly ground black pepper

Directions:

1. Preheat the oven to 425F.

2. In a bowl, combine the ghee, lemon zest, garlic, parsley, and lemon juice, season to taste with pepper and salt.

3. Put the fish into a greased baking dish. Season the fish to taste.

4. Pout the ghee mixture over the fish and top the fish with fresh slices of lemon; bake in the oven for about 12-25 minutes or until the fish is flaky.

5. Serve. If desired, top with fresh parsley.

Parmesan and Flaxseed Crusted Tilapia

Serves: 2

Net Carbs Per Serving: 1.5 grams

Prep. Time: 15 minutes

Cook Time: 7 minutes

Ingredients:

- 2 pieces (5-6 ounces) Tilapia filets

- 2 cloves garlic, minced or pressed

- 2 tablespoons ground flaxseed

- 2 tablespoons olive oil

- 2 tablespoons Parmesan Reggiano, finely shredded, OR regular parmesan cheese

- 4 tablespoons butter

- Sea salt

- White pepper

Directions:

1. Rinse and dry the tilapia fillets. Season with salt and pepper as desired. Set aside.

2. In an oven-safe dish or pan, add the olive oil and butter and heat over medium-high heat. Add the garlic and sauté until soft, but not browned.

3. Put the fish fillets into the pan, spooning the butter-garlic-oil mix over the fish. Cover and cook for about 4 minutes on medium heat until the fish flakes easily when tested with a fork.

4. In a small-sized bowl, combine the parmesan, flaxseed, and season with pepper and salt to taste. Cover the top of the fillets with the flaxseed mix, about 2 tablespoons each.

5. Spoon some of the butter-oil over the top to moisten.

6. Put the pan/dish in the broiler and broil for about 2-3 minutes or until the top is browned.

7. Serve with baby spinach or low carb dressing (I used

Newman's Light Italian Dressing).

Salmon Delight

Serves: 2

Net Carbs Per Serving:

Prep. Time: 15 minutes

Cook Time: 35-45 minutes

Ingredients:

- 1 pound salmon

- 1 tablespoon dried minced onion

- 1 teaspoon garlic, chopped

- 1/2 mayonnaise

- 1/2 teaspoon cayenne pepper

- 1/2 teaspoon paprika

- 1/2 teaspoon powdered mustard

- 1/4 teaspoon ground pepper

- 1/4 teaspoon kosher salt

Directions:

1. Put the salmon in a bowl. Toss and coat with the rest of the ingredients. Refrigerate for 1 hour to allow the flavors to intensify.

2. With the ski, side faced down, put the salmon on an aluminum foil sheet. Put remaining mixture on top of the salmon. Close the foil to seal the salmon, leaving a space for the steam.

3. Put in a preheated 350F oven and cook for about 35-45 minutes, depending on the salmon thickness.

Cheesy Salmon Loaf

Serves: 9

Net Carbs Per Serving:

Prep. Time: 10 minutes

Cook Time: 30 minutes

Ingredients:

- 1 can salmon

- 1 1/2 cup cheese, shredded

- 1 egg, beaten

- 1 tablespoon lemon juice

- 1/2 cup heavy cream

- 1/2 teaspoon pepper

- 1/2 teaspoon salt

- 2 tablespoons butter, melted

Directions:

1. Put all of the ingredients in a bowl and combine until mixed. Pour the mixture into greased bread pan.

2. Bake in a preheated 350F oven for 30 minutes.

Final Words

Thank you again for purchasing this book! I really hope this book is able to help you.

The next step is for you to **join our email newsletter** to receive updates on any upcoming new book releases or promotions. You can sign-up for free and as a bonus, you will also receive our "*7 Fitness Mistakes You Don't Know You're Making*" book! This bonus book breaks down many of the most common fitness mistakes and will demystify many of the complexities and science of getting into shape. Having all this fitness knowledge and science organized into an actionable step-by-step book will help you get started in the right direction in your fitness journey! To join our free email newsletter and grab your free book, please visit the link and signup: **www.hmwpublishing.com/gift**

Finally, if you enjoyed this book, then I would like to ask you for a favor, would you be kind enough to leave a review for this book? It would be greatly appreciated!

Thank you and good luck in your journey!

About the Co-Author

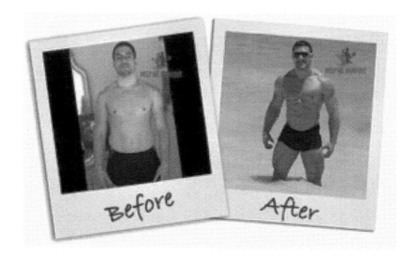

My name is George Kaplo; I'm a certified personal trainer from Montreal, Canada. I'll start off by saying I'm not the biggest guy you will ever meet and this has never really been my goal. In fact, I started working out to overcome my biggest insecurity when I was younger, which was my self-confidence. This was due to my height measuring only 5 foot 5 inches (168cm), it pushed me down to attempt anything I ever wanted to achieve in life. You may be going through some challenges right now, or you may simply want to get fit, and I can certainly relate.

For me personally, I was always kind of interested in the health & fitness world and wanted to gain some muscle due to the numerous bullying in my teenage years about my height and my overweight body. I figured I couldn't do anything about my height, but I sure can do something about how my body looked like. This was the beginning of my transformation journey. I had no idea where to start, but I just got started. I felt worried and afraid at times that other people would make fun of me for doing the exercises the wrong way. I always wished I had a friend that was next to me who was knowledgeable enough to help me get started and "show me the ropes."

After a lot of work, studying and countless trial and errors. Some people began to notice how I was getting more fit and how I was starting to form a keen interest in the topic. This led many friends and new faces to come to me and ask me for fitness advice. At first, it seemed odd when people asked me to help them get in shape. But what kept me going is when they started to see changes in their own body and told me it's the first time that they saw real results!

From there, more people kept coming to me, and it made me realize after so much reading and studying in this field that it did help me but it also allowed me to help others. I'm now a fully certified personal trainer and have trained numerous clients to date who have achieved amazing results.

Today, my brother Alex Kaplo (also a Certified Personal Trainer) and I own & operate this publishing venture, where we bring passionate and expert authors to write about health and fitness topics. We also run an online fitness website "HelpMeWorkout.com" and I would love to connect with by inviting you to visit the website on the following page and signing up to our e-mail newsletter (you will even get a free book).

Last but not least, if you are in the position I was once in and you want some guidance, don't hesitate and ask... I'll be there to help you out!

Your friend and coach,

George Kaplo
Certified Personal Trainer

Download another book for Free

I want to thank you for purchasing this book and offer you another book (just as long and valuable as this book), "Health & Fitness Mistakes You Don't Know You're Making", completely free.

Visit the link below to signup and receive it:

www.hmwpublishing.com/gift

In this book, I will break down the most common health & fitness mistakes, you are probably committing right now, and I will reveal how you can easily get in the best shape of your life!

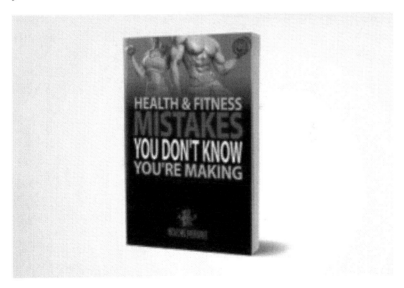

In addition to this valuable gift, you will also have an opportunity to get our new books for free, enter giveaways, and receive other valuable emails from me. Again, visit the link to sign up:

www.hmwpublishing.com/gift

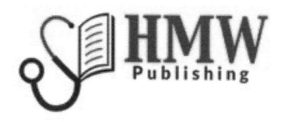

For more great books visit:

HMWPublishing.com

12-15
carbs from
Foundation
Vegies

5-8 other
carbs.

Breakfast

Made in the USA
Middletown, DE
29 February 2020